IMG Friendly Combined Med Peds Residency Programs List

With Comprehensive Match Selection Criteria and Programs Requirements

By

IMG Guide

And

Applicant Guide

Introduction

IMG Friendly Combined Medicine/Pediatrics Residency Programs

With Comprehensive Match Selection Criteria and Programs Requirements.

In Collaboration between the Applicant Guide and the IMG Guide we present to you the most complete and up-to-date IMG friendly Combined Med Peds residency programs list (Combined medicine pediatrics or Combined Med-Peds residency) with full match selection criteria and requirements for these programs. This book is essentially written for international medical graduates seeking residency in the US. The idea of writing this book came from our insight that many IMGs every year don't match because they don't know where to apply. Most of the time, they end applying to programs that don't have IMGs or those that don't match their criteria hence they end losing money with no interviews earned. The information was gathered from program directors, coordinators, chiefs, faculty and residents. It includes Programs names, Programs codes, States, Addresses, Phones, Faxes, Percentage of IMGs in the programs, Minimum USMLE Step 1 and Step 2 Score Requirements, Attempts on any step, CS requirement at time of application, USCE Requirements, Cut-Off time since graduation, Programs offering couple match and Visas Sponsored or accepted.

which is/are subject to change by/at the programs at any time. Although we did our best to get the most accurate information as much as possible from the program directors, coordinators, faculty and residents, however, you understand that by reading this book you are using the information here on your own responsibility.

Arkansas

University of Arkansas for Medical Sciences Combined Internal Med-Peds Residency Program

Specialty: Combined Internal Medicine-Pediatrics
Program name: University of Arkansas for Medical Sciences Program
Program code: 700-04-14-002
NRMP Code: 1018700C0
Program type: University-based
State: Arkansas
Address: University of Arkansas for Med Sciences, Internal Med H/S Office #634,
            4301 W Markham St, Little Rock, AR 72205-7199
Phone: (501) 686-5162
Fax: (501) 686-6001
Percentage of IMGs in the program: 25%
Minimum USMLE Step 1 Score Requirement: 210
Minimum USMLE Step 2 Score Requirement: 220
Attempts on any step: No limits set
CS required at time of application: Yes as well as ECFMG certificate
USCE Requirement: None
Cut-Off time since graduation: 7 years
Program offers couple match: Yes

Visas Sponsored or accepted: J1 visa and H1b visa

Florida

University of South Florida Morsani Combined Med/Peds Residency Program

Specialty: Combined Internal Medicine/Pediatrics
Program name: University of South Florida Morsani Program
Program code: 700-11-32-125
NRMP Code: 1109700C0
Program type: University-based
State: Florida
Address: University of South Florida College of Medicine, 5th Floor STC Room 5036,

2 Tampa General Circle, Tampa, FL 33606
Phone: (813) 259-8725
Fax: (813) 259-8792
Percentage of IMGs in the program: 15%
Minimum USMLE Step 1 Score Requirement: No limits set
Minimum USMLE Step 2 Score Requirement: No limits set
Attempts on any step: Maximum of two attempts one each step
CS required at time of application: No
USCE Requirement: None
Cut-Off time since graduation: 5 years
Program offers couple match: Yes
Visas Sponsored or accepted: J1 visa

Illinois

University of Illinois College of Medicine at Peoria Combined Med-Peds Residency Program

Specialty: Combined Internal Medicine/Pediatrics
Program name: University of Illinois College of Medicine at Peoria Program
Program code: 700-16-32-015

NRMP Code: 1175700C0
Program type: Community-based university affiliated hospital
State: Illinois
Address: OSF St Francis Medical Center, Med/Peds Program,
         530 NE Glen Oak Ave, Peoria, IL 61637
Phone: (309) 655-3863
Fax: (309) 655-4161
Percentage of IMGs in the program: 40%
Minimum USMLE Step 1 Score Requirement: No limits set
Minimum USMLE Step 2 Score Requirement: No limits set
Attempts on any step: Must pass on first attempt
CS required at time of application: Yes
USCE Requirement: None
Cut-Off time since graduation: 5 years unless clinically active
Program offers couple match: Yes
Visas Sponsored or accepted: J1 visa and H1b visa

Kansas

University of Kansas (Wichita) Combined Med-Peds Residency Program

Specialty: Combined Internal Medicine/Pediatrics
Program name: University of Kansas (Wichita) Program
Program code: 700-19-32-124
NRMP Code: 3054700C0
Program type: Community-based university affiliated hospital
State: Kansas
Address: University of Kansas School of Medicine-Wichita, Internal Medicine/Pediatrics, 550 N Hillside, Wichita, KS 67214
Phone: (316) 962-2212
Fax: (316) 962-7231
Percentage of IMGs in the program: 35%
Minimum USMLE Step 1 Score Requirement: No limits set
Minimum USMLE Step 2 Score Requirement: No limits set
Attempts on any step: Maximum of 2 attempts allowed on each step including the CS exam.
CS required at time of application: Yes including ECFMG certificate.
USCE Requirement: None
Cut-Off time since graduation: 5 years
Program offers couple match: Yes
Visas Sponsored or accepted: J1 visa

Louisiana

Louisiana State University (Shreveport) Combined Med-Peds Residency Program

Specialty: Combined Internal Medicine/Pediatrics
Program name: Louisiana State University (Shreveport) Program
Program code: 700-21-32-101
NRMP Code: 1232700C0
Program type: University-based
State: Louisiana
Address: LSU Health Science Center Shreveport, Department of Medicine,
          1501 Kings Hwy, Shreveport, LA 71130
Phone: (318) 675-5915
Fax: (318) 675-5988
Percentage of IMGs in the program: 60%
Minimum USMLE Step 1 Score Requirement: No limits set

Minimum USMLE Step 2 Score Requirement:
No limits set
Attempts on any step: Must pass on first attempt including CS exam
CS required at time of application: Yes
USCE Requirement: Yes
Cut-Off time since graduation: 5 years
Program offers couple match: Yes
Visas Sponsored or accepted: J1 visa

Louisiana State University Combined Med-Peds Residency Program

Specialty: Combined Internal Medicine/Pediatrics
Program name: Louisiana State University Program
Program code: 700-21-14-022
Program type: University-based
State: Louisiana
Address: LSU Health Science Center New Orleans, Box T4M-2 4th Floor Room 441A,
          1542 Tulane Ave, New Orleans, LA 70112
Phone: (504) 568-3792
Fax: (504) 568-2127
Percentage of IMGs in the program: 85%
Minimum USMLE Step 1 Score Requirement: 210

Minimum USMLE Step 2 Score Requirement: 210
Attempts on any step: Must pass on first attempt
CS required at time of application: Yes including ECFMG Certificate
USCE Requirement: Yes
Cut-Off time since graduation: 2 years
Program offers couple match: Yes
Visas Sponsored or accepted: J1 visa

Michigan

William Beaumont Hospital Combined Med-Peds Residency Program

Specialty: Combined Internal Medicine/Pediatrics
Program name: William Beaumont Hospital Program
Program code: 700-25-32-033
NRMP Code: 1978700C0

Program type: Community-based university affiliated hospital
State: Michigan
Address: William Beaumont Hospital, Med/Peds Program,
          3601 W 13 Mile Rd, Royal Oak, MI 48073-6769
Phone: (248) 551-6489
Fax: (248) 551-8880
Percentage of IMGs in the program: 50%
Minimum USMLE Step 1 Score Requirement: 210
Minimum USMLE Step 2 Score Requirement: 210
Attempts on any step: No limits set
CS required at time of application: No
USCE Requirement: None
Cut-Off time since graduation: No limits set
Program offers couple match: Yes
Visas Sponsored or accepted: J1 visa and H1b visa

Western Michigan University School of Medicine Combined Med-Peds Residency Program

Specialty: Combined Internal Medicine/Pediatrics
Program name: Western Michigan University School of Medicine Program

Program code: 700-25-14-089
NRMP Code: 1314700C0
Program type: Community-based university affiliated hospital
State: Michigan
Address: Western Michigan University School of Medicine, Med/Peds Program
            1000 Oakland Dr, Kalamazoo, MI 49008
Phone: (269) 337-6353
Fax: (269) 337-4262
Percentage of IMGs in the program: 20%
Minimum USMLE Step 1 Score Requirement: 225
Minimum USMLE Step 2 Score Requirement: 225
Attempts on any step: Must pass on first attempt
CS required at time of application: No
USCE Requirement: None
Cut-Off time since graduation: 5 years unless clinically active like in residency or clinical practice
Program offers couple match: Yes
Visas Sponsored or accepted: J1 visa and H1b visa

Hurley Medical Center/Michigan State University Combined Med-Peds Residency Program

Specialty: Combined Internal Medicine/Pediatrics
Program name: Hurley Medical Center/Michigan State University Program
Program code: 700-25-32-030
NRMP Code: 1307700C0
Program type: Community-based university affiliated hospital
State: Michigan
Address: Hurley Medical Center, Combined Med-Peds Education 3AW,
　　　　One Hurley Plaza, Flint, MI 48503
Phone: (810) 262-9283
Fax: (810) 262-9736
Percentage of IMGs in the program: 10%
Minimum USMLE Step 1 Score Requirement: 206
Minimum USMLE Step 2 Score Requirement: 206
Attempts on any step: No limits set
CS required at time of application: Yes as well as ECFMG certificate
USCE Requirement: None
Cut-Off time since graduation: 5 years unless clinically active as residency or clinical practice.
Program offers couple match: Yes

Visas Sponsored or accepted: J1 visa and H1b visa

Missouri

St. Louis University School of Medicine Combined Med/Peds Residency Program

Specialty: Combined Internal Medicine/Pediatrics
Program name: St Louis University School of Medicine Program
Program code: 700-28-14-037
Program type: University-based
State: Missouri
Address: St Louis University School of Medicine, Department of Internal Medicine,
        1402 S Grand Blvd, St Louis, MO 63104
Phone: (314) 577-8762
Fax: (314) 268-5108
Percentage of IMGs in the program: 40%
Minimum USMLE Step 1 Score Requirement: 212

Minimum USMLE Step 2 Score Requirement: 212
Attempts on any step: Must pass on first attempt
CS required at time of application: No
USCE Requirement: Yes
Cut-Off time since graduation: 5 years
Program offers couple match: Yes
Visas Sponsored or accepted: J1 visa and H1b visa

Nebraska

University of Nebraska Medical Center College of Medicine Combined Med-Peds Residency Program

Specialty: Combined Internal Medicine/Pediatrics
Program name: University of Nebraska Medical Center College of Medicine Program
Program code: 700-30-14-136
NRMP Code: 1376700C0
Program type: University-based
State: Nebraska

Address: University of Nebraska Medical Center, Department of Internal Medicine Education,

982055 Nebraska Med Center, Omaha, NE 68198-2055
Phone: (402) 559-7792
Fax: (402) 559-9385
Percentage of IMGs in the program: 15%
Minimum USMLE Step 1 Score Requirement: 205
Minimum USMLE Step 2 Score Requirement: 205
Attempts on any step: Must pass on first attempt
CS required at time of application: No
USCE Requirement: None
Cut-Off time since graduation: No limits set
Program offers couple match: Yes
Visas Sponsored or accepted: J1 visa and H1b visa

New Jersey

Newark Beth Israel Medical Center Combined Med-Peds Residency Program

Specialty: Combined Internal Medicine/Pediatrics
Program name: Newark Beth Israel Medical Center Program
Program code: 700-33-32-041
State: New Jersey
Address: Newark Beth Israel Medical Center, Medicine-Pediatrics,
        201 Lyons Ave, Newark, NJ 07112
Phone: (973) 926-4949
Fax: (973) 923-2441
Percentage of IMGs in the program: 40%
Minimum USMLE Step 1 Score Requirement: 210
Minimum USMLE Step 2 Score Requirement: 210
Attempts on any step: No limits set
CS required at time of application: No
USCE Requirement: None
Cut-Off time since graduation: 2 years
Program offers couple match: Yes
Visas Sponsored or accepted: No visa

UMDNJ-New Jersey Medical School Combined Med-Peds Residency Program

Specialty: Combined Internal Medicine/Pediatrics

Program name: Rutgers New Jersey Medical School Program
Program code: 700-33-32-040
NRMP Code: 1398700C0
Program type: University-based
State: New Jersey
Address: Rutgers New Jersey Medical School, UH I-247,

150 Bergen St, Newark, NJ 07103
Phone: (973) 972-6056
Fax: (973) 972-3129
Percentage of IMGs in the program: 30%
Minimum USMLE Step 1 Score Requirement: No limits set
Minimum USMLE Step 2 Score Requirement: No limits set
Attempts on any step: No limits set
CS required at time of application: No
USCE Requirement: None
Cut-Off time since graduation: No limits set
Program offers couple match: Yes
Visas Sponsored or accepted: J1 visa

New York

SUNY at Stony Brook Combined Med-Peds Residency Program

Specialty: Combined Internal Medicine/Pediatrics
Program name: SUNY at Stony Brook Program
Program code: 700-35-32-093
NRMP Code: 2919700C0
Program type: University-based
State: New York
Address: SUNY Stony Brook University, Internal Medicine/Pediatrics Program,
 HSC T-11 040, Stony Brook, NY 11794-8111
Phone: (631) 444-2020
Percentage of IMGs in the program: 20%
Minimum USMLE Step 1 Score Requirement: No limits set
Minimum USMLE Step 2 Score Requirement: No limits set
Attempts on any step: Must pass on first attempt including CS exam
CS required at time of application: Yes
USCE Requirement: None
Cut-Off time since graduation: 10 years
Program offers couple match: Yes
Visas Sponsored or accepted: J1 visa

Albany Medical Center Combined Med-Peds Residency Program

Specialty: Combined Internal Medicine/Pediatrics
Program name: Albany Medical Center Program
Program code: 700-35-14-044
NRMP Code: 1414700C0
Program type: University-based
State: New York
Address: Albany Medical Center, Internal Medicine/Pediatrics Program,
724 Watervliet-Shaker Rd, Latham, NY 12110
Phone: (518) 262-7585
Fax: (518) 262-7505
Percentage of IMGs in the program: 20%
Minimum USMLE Step 1 Score Requirement: No limits set
Minimum USMLE Step 2 Score Requirement: No limits set
Attempts on any step: Must pass on first attempt
CS required at time of application: No
USCE Requirement: Yes
Cut-Off time since graduation: 5 years unless clinically active as in residency or practice.
Program offers couple match: Yes
Visas Sponsored or accepted: J1 visa

University at Buffalo Combined Med-Peds Residency Program

Specialty: Combined Internal Medicine/Pediatrics
Program name: University at Buffalo Program
Program code: 700-35-32-049
NRMP Code: 3099700C0
Program type: Community-based university affiliated hospital
State: New York
Address: Women and Children's Hospital Buffalo, Division of Internal Medicine-Pediatrics,
          300 Linwood Ave, Buffalo, NY 14209
Phone: (716) 961-9412
Fax: (716) 961-9403
Percentage of IMGs in the program: 40%
Minimum USMLE Step 1 Score Requirement: 205
Minimum USMLE Step 2 Score Requirement: 205
Attempts on any step: Must pass on first attempt
CS required at time of application: No
USCE Requirement: Yes
Cut-Off time since graduation: 2 years
Program offers couple match: Yes
Visas Sponsored or accepted: J1 visa

North Carolina

Vidant Medical Center/East Carolina University Combined Med-Peds Residency Program

Specialty: Combined Internal Medicine/Pediatrics
Program name: Vidant Medical Center/East Carolina University Program
Program code: 700-36-32-057
NRMP Code: 3057700C0
Program type: University-based
State: North Carolina
Address: Brody School of Medicine ECU, PCMH-MA 307,

600 Moye Blvd, Greenville, NC 27834
Phone: (252) 744-3961
Fax: (252) 744-4688
Percentage of IMGs in the program: 15%
Minimum USMLE Step 1 Score Requirement: No limits set
Minimum USMLE Step 2 Score Requirement: No limits set
Attempts on any step: No limits set
CS required at time of application: No
USCE Requirement: None
Cut-Off time since graduation: 3 years
Program offers couple match: Yes
Visas Sponsored or accepted: J1 visa

Duke University Hospital Combined Med-Peds Residency Program

Specialty: Combined Internal Medicine/Pediatrics
Program name: Duke University Hospital Program
Program code: 700-36-14-056
NRMP Code:
Program type:
State: North Carolina
Address: Duke University Medical Center, Department of Medicine-Pediatrics,
          Box 3127, Durham, NC 27710
Phone: (919) 681-3009
Fax: (919) 681-5825
Percentage of IMGs in the program: 5%
Minimum USMLE Step 1 Score Requirement: No limits set
Minimum USMLE Step 2 Score Requirement: No limits set
Attempts on any step: No limits set
CS required at time of application: Yes including ECFMG certificate
USCE Requirement: None
Cut-Off time since graduation: No limits set
Program offers couple match: Yes
Visas Sponsored or accepted: J1 visa

Ohio

Ohio State University Hospital Combined Med-Peds Residency Program

Specialty: Combined Internal Medicine/Pediatrics
Program name: Ohio State University Hospital Program
Program code: 700-38-14-063
NRMP Code: 1566700C0
Program type: University-based
State: Ohio
Address: Nationwide Children's Hospital, Rm ED-650A,
 700 Children's Dr, Columbus, OH 43205
Phone: (614) 722-0417
Fax: (614) 722-6132
Percentage of IMGs in the program: 0% (occasionally 1 resident)
Minimum USMLE Step 1 Score Requirement: No limits set
Minimum USMLE Step 2 Score Requirement: No limits set
Attempts on any step: No limits set
CS required at time of application: Yes
USCE Requirement: Yes
Cut-Off time since graduation: 5 years

Program offers couple match: Yes
Visas Sponsored or accepted: J1 visa and H1b visa

Case Western Reserve University/University Hospitals Case Medical Center Combined Med-Peds Residency Program

Specialty: Combined Internal Medicine/Pediatrics
Program name: Case Western Reserve University/University Hospitals Case Medical Center Program
Program code: 700-38-32-121
NRMP Code: 1552700C0
Program type: University-based
State: Ohio
Address: University Hospitals Case Medical Center, Lakeside 1507,
          11100 Euclid Ave, Cleveland, OH 44106-6055
Phone: (216) 844-8431
Fax: (216) 844-7497
Percentage of IMGs in the program: 65%
Minimum USMLE Step 1 Score Requirement: No limits set
Minimum USMLE Step 2 Score Requirement: No limits set
Attempts on any step: No limits set

CS required at time of application: No
USCE Requirement: None
Cut-Off time since graduation: 3 years
Program offers couple match: Yes
Visas Sponsored or accepted: J1 visa

Case Western Reserve University (MetroHealth) Combined Med-Peds Residency Program

Specialty: Combined Internal Medicine/Pediatrics
Program name: Case Western Reserve University (MetroHealth) Program
Program code: 700-38-32-061
NRMP Code: 1553700C0
Program type: University-based
State: Ohio
Address: MetroHealth Medical Center, Internal Medicine-Pediatrics H574,
        2500 MetroHealth Dr, Cleveland, OH 44109-1998
Phone: (216) 778-2882
Fax: (216) 778-1384
Percentage of IMGs in the program: 35%
Minimum USMLE Step 1 Score Requirement: 210
Minimum USMLE Step 2 Score Requirement: 210

Attempts on any step: Must pass on first attempt including CS exam
CS required at time of application: No
USCE Requirement: None
Cut-Off time since graduation: 5 years
Program offers couple match: Yes
Visas Sponsored or accepted: J1 visa and H1b visa

Oklahoma

University of Oklahoma College of Medicine-Tulsa Combined Med-Peds Residency Program

Specialty: Combined Internal Medicine/Pediatrics
Program name: University of Oklahoma College of Medicine-Tulsa Program
Program code: 700-39-32-067
State: Oklahoma
Address: University of Oklahoma Coll of Med-Tulsa, Sect of Med/Pediatrics #3G06,
4502 E 41st St, Tulsa, OK 74135-2512
Phone: (918) 660-3395
Fax: (918) 660-3444
Percentage of IMGs in the program: 25%

Minimum USMLE Step 1 Score Requirement:
205
Minimum USMLE Step 2 Score Requirement:
205
Attempts on any step: No limits set
CS required at time of application: No
USCE Requirement: None
Cut-Off time since graduation: No limits set
Program offers couple match: Yes
Visas Sponsored or accepted: J1 visa and H1b
visa

University of Oklahoma Health Sciences Center Combined Med-Peds Residency Program

Specialty: Combined Internal
Medicine/Pediatrics
Program name: University of Oklahoma Health
Sciences Center Program
Program code: 700-39-32-090
NRMP Code: 1588700C0
Program type: University-based
State: Oklahoma
Address: Children's Hospital Oklahoma City, A2
14000,
          1200 Children's Ave, Oklahoma City,
OK 73104
Phone: (405) 271-4417
Fax: (405) 271-2920

Percentage of IMGs in the program: 60%
Minimum USMLE Step 1 Score Requirement:
No limits set
Minimum USMLE Step 2 Score Requirement:
No limits set
Attempts on any step: No limits set
CS required at time of application: Yes
including ECFMG certificate
USCE Requirement: None
Cut-Off time since graduation: 3 years
Program offers couple match: Yes
Visas Sponsored or accepted: J1 visa

Pennsylvania

Penn State University/Milton S Hershey Medical Center Combined Med-Peds Residency Program

Specialty: Combined Internal
Medicine/Pediatrics
Program name: Penn State Milton S Hershey
Medical Center Program
Program code: 700-41-32-081
NRMP Code: 1617700C0
Program type: University-based
State: Pennsylvania

Address: Milton S Hershey Medical Center, PO Box 850 MC H085,
500 University Dr, Hershey, PA 17033-0850
Phone: (717) 531-8899
Fax: (717) 531-0856
Percentage of IMGs in the program: 10%
Minimum USMLE Step 1 Score Requirement: No limits set
Minimum USMLE Step 2 Score Requirement: No limits set
Attempts on any step: No limits set
CS required at time of application: No
USCE Requirement: None
Cut-Off time since graduation: 2 years
Program offers couple match: Yes
Visas Sponsored or accepted: J1 visa

Geisinger Health System Combined Med-Peds Residency Program

Specialty: Combined Internal Medicine/Pediatrics
Program name: Geisinger Health System Program
Program code: 700-41-14-068
NRMP Code: 1608700C0
Program type: Community-based university affiliated hospital
State: Pennsylvania

Address: Geisinger Medical Center, MC 01-38,
          100 N Academy Ave, Danville, PA
17822-0138
Phone: (570) 271-6520
Fax: (570) 214-6354
Percentage of IMGs in the program: 30%
Minimum USMLE Step 1 Score Requirement:
No limits set
Minimum USMLE Step 2 Score Requirement:
No limits set
Attempts on any step: Must pass on first
attempt
CS required at time of application: No
USCE Requirement: None
Cut-Off time since graduation: No limits set
Program offers couple match: Yes
Visas Sponsored or accepted: J1 visa and H1b
visa

Tennessee

University of Tennessee Combined Med-Peds Residency Program

Specialty: Combined Internal
Medicine/Pediatrics

Program name: University of Tennessee Program
Program code: 700-47-32-071
NRMP Code: 1844700C0
Program type: University-based
State: Tennessee
Address: University of Tennessee Medical Center, Room H316,
          956 Court Ave, Memphis, TN 38163
Phone: (901) 448-3714
Fax: (901) 448-7836
Percentage of IMGs in the program: 8%
Minimum USMLE Step 1 Score Requirement: 210
Minimum USMLE Step 2 Score Requirement: 210
Attempts on any step: Must pass on first attempt
CS required at time of application: No
USCE Requirement: Yes, 3 months
Cut-Off time since graduation: 5 years unless clinically active as in residency or practice
Program offers couple match: Yes
Visas Sponsored or accepted: J1 visa

West Virginia

West Virginia University Combined Med-Peds Residency Program

Specialty: Combined Internal Medicine/Pediatrics
Program name: West Virginia University Program
Program code: 700-55-32-080
Program type: University-based
State: West Virginia
Address: West Virginia University School of Medicine, Department of Pediatrics,
                PO Box 9214, Morgantown, WV 26506-9214
Phone: (304) 293-1224
Fax: (304) 293-1216
Percentage of IMGs in the program: 20%
Minimum USMLE Step 1 Score Requirement: 205
Minimum USMLE Step 2 Score Requirement: 205
Attempts on any step: No limits set
CS required at time of application: Yes
USCE Requirement: None
Cut-Off time since graduation: 5 years
Program offers couple match: Yes
Visas Sponsored or accepted: J1 visa

Charleston Area Medical Center/West Virginia University (Charleston Division) Combined Med-Peds Residency Program

Specialty: Combined Internal Medicine/Pediatrics
Program name: Charleston Area Medical Center/West Virginia University (Charleston Division) Program
Program code: 700-55-14-078
NRMP Code: 1902700C0
Program type: Community-based university affiliated hospital
State: West Virginia
Address: Charleston Area Medical Center, Medicine/Pediatrics Program Ste 104,
830 Pennsylvania Ave, Charleston, WV 25302
Phone: (304) 388-1589
Fax: (304) 388-2926
Percentage of IMGs in the program: 25%
Minimum USMLE Step 1 Score Requirement: No limits set
Minimum USMLE Step 2 Score Requirement: No limits set
Attempts on any step: Must pass from first attempt
CS required at time of application: Yes including ECFMG certificate

USCE Requirement: None
Cut-Off time since graduation: No limits set
Program offers couple match: Yes
Visas Sponsored or accepted: J1 visa

Wisconsin

Marshfield Clinic-St Joseph Hospital Combined Med-Peds Residency Program

Specialty: Combined Internal Medicine/Pediatrics
Program name: Marshfield Clinic-St Joseph's Hospital Program
Program code: 700-56-14-109
NRMP Code: 1780700C0
Program type: Community-based university affiliated hospital
State: Wisconsin
Address: Marshfield Clinic, Med-Peds Program 1F2,
      1000 N Oak Ave, Marshfield, WI 54449
Phone: (800) 541-2895   Ext: 93141
Fax: (715) 389-3142
Percentage of IMGs in the program: 60%

Minimum USMLE Step 1 Score Requirement: 210
Minimum USMLE Step 2 Score Requirement: 210
Attempts on any step: No limits set
CS required at time of application: Yes including ECFMG certificate
USCE Requirement: None
Cut-Off time since graduation: 5 years unless clinically active as in residency or practice
Program offers couple match: Yes
Visas Sponsored or accepted: J1 visa and H1b visa

Contents

Please take 1 minute to write a review and rate our book on Amazon. We wish you a successful match. Thank you for buying our book.

If you have any questions please email us at applicantguide@yahoo.com

IMG Guide
&
Applicant Guide

www.imgguide.com
www.applicantguide.com